Light the fire inside
you...

With all your might stop
smoking.

Read books about it.

Disgust yourself by
smoking and putting out
your cigarette.

Most of all, think of something horrible that makes you stop.

It will kill you.

Life is short.

My dad died from lung cancer.

I assure you it is a painful sad way to die.

Ignite your childhood imagination inside you.

Remember running on the playground.

Remind yourself of how many days you have missed work.

It is uncool to smoke.

You will use it as a stress relief.

It is not a stress relief.

It does not go well with alcohol.

Light the fire inside inside you.

Be the person you were meant to be.

Write or journal about it.

Help friends quit.
Sip water all day if you have to every time you want a cigarette.

Replace a negative with a positive.

Try meditation.

Listen to music.

Squeeze a ball.

Try chewing gummy
bears or sucking mints.

Come up with a system
that works for you.
Take a cold shower.

Eat healthy carrots or cucumbers every time you want a cigarette.

Don't use vapors.

Quit using your own vices.

Mostly , believe you can quit.

You can't stop unless you want to.

I stopped because I don't want to die like my father.

It is awful to stop.

You get moody.

You don't want to go out to bars.

You watch a lot of movies.

The first month is the worst.

You will cheat.

Then, you will eventually get angry at yourself for cheating.

I stopped and have been
a non-smoker for ten
years.

It was the hardest thing
I ever did.

No excuses.

You need to quit.

Make a positive example for your children.

Make a promise to yourself.

Day by day.

It will get better.

You are strong.

You are a fighter.

Nicotine is bad.

Light the fire of inspiration to quit smoking in your neighborhood.

Start a group to quit smoking in your drive way. Everyone needs support.

Be brave.

Be strong.

Smoking is not a good vice.

Once you quit you will feel so free.

Free from guilt.

Replace it will
something healthy like
yoga or meditation.

Play basketball.

Reward yourself in a
positive way.

Remember once you
stop smoking.

You can accomplish anything.

Break your boundaries in a safe way.

Fly somewhere new.

Breath better.

Smell better.

Begin again and help
others.

You can do anything you
put your mind to.

Visualize you have
stopped smoking.

Realize every breath is
worth fighting for.

Living on oxygen is no fun.

Dying young is not inevitable.

You still have great things to do.

People to share your story with.

Family members to
forgive.

Children to help.

Love to give.

Fences to mend.

People to face.

It is a chapter you need
to close in your life.

The patch helped me but it took about eight weeks.

Then, it was my will power that finally made me never want to lite up again.

Use your imagination to conquer your habit.

Lie in bed and pull the covers over your head.

Realize it is an addiction and you will beat it.

Remember everything that is hard in life is worth it. It helps us regain belief in ourselves.

I never thought I could quit.

I smoked two packs a day.

I was sick all the time.

I choose to live and hope you do too.

Choose a method that works for you.

Read as many books as
you can.

Look at nasty pictures of
your lungs.

Put the light out in your
cigarette.

Learn from it and grow
from it.

You can accomplish this.

I believe you can because I did.

Change your routine.

If you need coffee and a smoke.

Have a smoothie and a banana.

Try anything you can within reason to stop smoking.

Celebrate with your friends and family.

Achieve this goal for you and no one else.

It will be the best decision of your life.

I can't make you quit. I
can just tell you it is
worth it.

Eventually, you will have
a coffee without a
smoke.

You will eat dinner and
not need a smoke.

You will discover new
things about yourself.

Nothing is handed to us.

Life is full of desires and temptations.

Refuse to give in.

Be the person you were destined to be.

Use an elastic band to remind you not to

smoke. If you snap the elastic band on your wrist every time you want a smoke it might help.

Smoking is not for you.

Set your mind free.

Free to write.

Free to paint.

Start a podcast to help others.

Engage in helping others.

That is why we are here.

Not to judge.

We all fail.

We all overcome
imperfections.

When your guided by
your heart your mind
starts to kick in.

Just do it so you can say
you did it.

Make a plan a stick to it.

Walk.

Dream.

Begin each day with
new hope.

This will not be easy.

It will take time.

It is worth all your time
and effort.

Become a role model.

Lead and be guided by something you want to leave behind.

We all have useless information that might help someone else.

Open up again.

Climb those mountains.

Tare down those
stereotypes.

Embrace what life has
thrown at you.

Be brave enough to
stifle through the crap.
The excuses we tell
ourselves to stay
smokers.

Destiny is yours for the making.

Even dancing takes steps.

Learn your new steps.

Butt out literally.

Butting out your smoke can perhaps put you on your next path.

Bring light to others.

Shine through your
hardships.

Press on forward
because that is the only
choice you have.

You have a gift and you
need to believe that.

We are all good at
something find out what
that is?

Dig yourself out of the
hole with your shovel...

We never know how
long we have.

Just get through one
day.

Then, the next day.

Then, the next day.

You are much braver then you thought.

You will see.

You will be the best version of yourself a non-smoker.

Be brave-butt out.

Light the fire inside you not the fire for your cigarette.